Runner For Life

Stories and Running Tips From

The Streaking Runner

Copyright 2012
ISBN: 978-1469937847

Acknowledgments

Thanks to my wonderful husband who understands me completely! Thanks for your love and support in all that I do. Thanks for understanding that my run for the day happens – even if nothing else does that day. And, thanks for the years of "stuff holding" at races, bearing with me while I get my run in on vacations, taking me on our "running vacations" and understanding that the night before a long run or race means pizza or spaghetti! I love you with all my heart!

Thanks to my parents who instilled in me the independence that I have and the sense that it's alright to be myself in all I do. Thanks for your support in my running and in everything I do!

Thanks to all my running buddies through the years. Jackie Janice Murphy – my college "RP" (running partner). Lee Scruggs, Dan Withrow, Randy Mullens – the early years and the ones who made me a streaker. Dan Wright and Dave Oliver , thanks for getting me through those "Runner's World" days and being my running "besties" for so long!

Table of Contents

Introduction

To begin with, this is not a book about naked running. This is about my life as a running "streaker". A streaker in running means that you have run a certain amount of time without missing a day. Probably not as exciting as naked running, but it is to me!

In my case, I have not missed a day of running since November 20, 1985. This book talks about my running during those years – the ups and downs, the funny stories and more.

I'll also share some information with you that will keep you on the roads for many years – if you are already a runner. If not, then I'll give you some reasons why you should start a running program.

It's hard to express how much running has meant to me. It's kept me in pretty good shape, in good health and just an overall sense of well-being. My Dad says that I was always "pretty high-strung", so running helps keep me on an even keel. Running is so great for working through problems and putting life into perspective. Like I say, running is cheaper than a therapist!

Not everyone is cut out to be a streaker. But, it works for me. I hope you enjoy the stories of my running journey!

Chapter 1 – The Beginning

November 20, 1985, is an important day in my running. That's the day that I became a streaker. But, my running began long before that.

My Dad and I used to go running when I was younger. He measured off 1½ miles around our neighborhood that was our route. Now, this was in the late '60's – early 70's. Not a lot was heard about running and in a small town – pretty non-existent. No running stores, no technical clothing, not even running shoes. And, truthfully, no other runners.

But, that didn't stop us. After dinner, I'd pull on my P.F. Flyers and away we'd go! My dad and I out on the road. He'd look at his watch (also no running watch) and make note of the time that we were gone. Daddy even wrote down the time that it took us to run. My first running log!

I'm sure we weren't fast – but it was fun being out with my Dad! I'm an only child and these times with Daddy were really special. Truthfully, I'm not sure that I really enjoyed it that much – but I was out with my Dad, and that was all that mattered!

I'm not sure how long a time that we kept up our running. Sometimes I wonder what would have happened if I had kept it up then. Would I have been faster, would I have been better?

Or would I have given up on it later and not gone back. I'll never know – but, I believe that it worked out the way it was supposed to.

Chapter 2 – Not A High School Athlete

Many people think that they have to be athletic their whole life in order to be a runner. Well, I am living proof of that NOT being the case.

Now, when I was a kid, I was a tomboy. I played ball with the neighborhood boys, I rode my bike all the time, etc. So, being wimpy was not the case, but I was never what you would call athletic. I was small boned and had skinny arms.

Do you remember Red Rover? Just the name still makes me cringe. It's a game played during Phys Ed were you pick teams and then line up across from each other. You grab onto the person's arm that is next to you. The object is for someone for the one team to run as hard as they can toward the line made by the opposing team and break through the arm link.

First of all, I was always one of the last ones chosen for a team. Always great for a grade-schooler's confidence. Then, I was always the first person that the opposing team tried to get through. And, the next, and if I was still holding on, the next. It's a wonder I made it through school without a broken arm.

In Junior High School, my Physical Education teacher actually gave me a few B's. OK, more than a few. In P.E.! Who gets B's in P.E.? I was a straight A student with some B's in P.E. I never thought that I was any worse than some of the students who got A's, but who knows. In Senior High, I decided that I'd had enough of the whole Phys Ed thing. Luckily, if you were in band, you didn't need to take P.E., so I was off the hook.

Now that I've run several marathons, I want to go up to my Junior High Phys Ed teacher sometime and tell her......., OK, I won't go there! But, you get my point. Just because a person is not known as athletic when they are younger, doesn't mean that they can't turn into an athlete. I really do consider myself to be one now.

Chapter 3 – Starting Again

After that, I didn't run again until I was in college. When I was a sophomore, my best college friend, Jackie, and I decided to start running. She and I called each other "RP" for running partner – which we still call each other today. We had a two-fold purpose for starting to run.

First of all, I had put on.....well......we'll just say several pounds the first 2 years of college. So, I figured that running would be a great way to get them off. My friend had another purpose in mind. She was trying to catch the eye of a member of the cross country team. Well, the story ends well. I'm still running and she is still married to the cross country runner!

Running then was so simple. Technical running clothing was still something that we knew nothing about. I figured that you had to be a member of a team to get "running" clothes. We wore cotton gym shorts or any pair of shorts we could and a cotton tee shirt. Running bra? Nope, just our regular, wear every day bra.

We measured our time by a good old Timex watch – once again, not a running one, just a regular that had a band that would not disintegrate with sweat. I actually think that I still have that watch somewhere.

I remember running in the cooler weather in a pair of jeans, my junior high band jacket, a wool scarf around my neck and wool mittens. Boy, have I come a long way since then. But, I wanted to run, I didn't have access to anywhere to buy running clothes, so I made do.

Luckily, I was able to get a decent pair of running shoes. My parents owned a retail clothing store and we carried Converse tennis shoes. I talked my Dad into ordering me a pair of running shoes. I thought I was in heaven the first time I put them on! Converse was my shoe of choice for many years after that. At the time, they made a great shoe!

When we first started running, we ran around the track at college before we ventured out on the roads. We'd run as far as we could, walk some and then run some until we reached a mile. Every time we ran, we'd try to go a little farther with our running than the time before. The first time we ran a whole mile – you'd have thought we discovered America or something. We were SO excited! It was a great way to get started with running – and that's how I recommend to everyone to start.

Running then was definitely different than it is now. Believe me, there were very few of us out there. But, we had fun – and sometimes I miss the simplicity of those runs.

Chapter 4 – My First Race

In my hometown, there is an Osteopathic School of Medicine. For many years, they sponsored a 10K (6.2 miles) road race the first week-end in May. This was a great race and I'm really sorry that they stopped having it.

Anyway, Jackie and I had been running for several months now. So, we figured it was time to run a race. Since the Osteopathic School race was coming up, road trip to our first race was scheduled!

I remember filling out that first race entry blank. Once it was sent in the mail – I felt like such the "real runner"! I was going to run a race – that was the ultimate! And, they were going to give me a free t-shirt. How cool was that!

Just a side note on the t-shirt for that race. They had a really cool logo that you knew whenever you saw that shirt just what race it was from. Every year they changed the color, but the front logo remained the same. I loved that shirt – and I have several of them!

Jackie and I were so excited to be doing a race. We ran with a new vengeance – we had to be ready to run 6 miles. And, of course, we had to look good doing it.

So, race week-end was finally here. We traveled to my hometown and unloaded at my parents' house. Then, it was time to pick up our race packet – and get that first race t-shirt! There we were with other runners and we were part of the crowd. We were so excited!

It was hard to sleep that night – but we did and were up fairly early. We dressed for the race - in our non-technical white gym shorts and our race t-shirts. (OK, now I know that most people don't wear the race t-shirt of the current race to run the race – but we didn't care. We were proud to wear them!)

This race was a point to point, so we had to be bussed to the starting line. Once again, on the bus, here we were with a bunch of other runners on the bus and definitely feeling part of the running family.

After a little wait, the gun went off – and so did we! Our first race! The course was a rolling road through some picturesque farmland. The finish was a downhill and then flat to the finish line – which was downtown. It was SO neat to have a great finish with a big crowd there cheering you on!

Jackie and I went on to run several more races together before college was over. But we will never forget the fun and the thrill of that first one!

Chapter 5 – The Streak Begins

I didn't start out with the idea that I was going to become a streaker. After college was a busy time. I had started working full time for my parents helping them run our retail department store. A couple of years after college, I got married to my soul mate – life was good.

I had been running on and off since college, been running a few races, but not real serious about it.

I saw a notice about some local runners that were wanting to start a running club in our town, so I went to the first meeting. I met some wonderful people who I am still friends with today.

We had so much fun. We'd all pack in someone's car and head 45 minutes to an hour on Saturdays for a race. Our running group also started another race in our town. It was a great time.

Then, one day, talk started about streaks. Being an only child – and a redhead – I can sometimes be a little competitive. (Remember, my Dad says I'm a little "high-strung"). Anyway, I was intrigued and there was no way streaks were going to happen without me!

I did a little researching on running streaks. Some people consider different things to qualify, but in my book, it has to be at least a mile. Now, most days, my run is more than a mile. I actually consider 2 miles to be a rest day – but that's just me. And, the mile days come when I'm really feeling sick – which luckily have been few and far between. (My health is another bi-product of my streaking – in my opinion!).

So, November 20, 1985, was the day the streak began. I'm not sure if my fellow streakers are still going, but I am. And, I feel like I'm a better and more motivated runner for it!

Chapter 6 – Races/Medals/Beating Rivals

Races were always fun to go to. If there was a race anywhere within an hour of me, I was there – with a group or not. The distance of the race didn't matter to us. We'd do anything from 5K's to 10K's to 15-milers.

As I got a little faster, along came the age group awards. Nowadays, winning an age group award is not as important as it once was – but I still get excited when I do. But, there was a time when it was. (Keep in mind my competitive nature).

Awards are usually given to the first three overall runners and the first 3 finishers in a certain age group – divided up male and female. The usual age group award is a medal on a ribbon. When the race was over, everyone sits around waiting to see who won the awards. It was such a thrill whenever you're name is called and you get to go up in front of everyone and pick up a medal!

You also get to see who the others are that you're competing against in your age group. There are always a couple of them that are "super competitive"! There was always this one runner who usually beat me. One race, I went by her with about a mile to go. I said the usual, "hey" as I went by. Well, then, a few yards later, here she came blasting by me – but I could tell she was breathing really hard. So, I pushed a little more, got by her and stayed ahead of her to the finish line.

I can't even remember if I won an age group award that day – it was just the satisfaction of beating someone who had always beat me! And couldn't stand the fact that I finished ahead of her!

Speaking of that, in my group of runners that I ran with in my home town, the guys usually beat me. By usually, I mean all the time. Not by much, but all the time. One race, I was coming up on the finish line and I could see one of the guys just a little ahead of me. OK, I thought, here is my chance. I kicked it into another gear and passed him.

I was so excited! I had finally beaten one of the guys. Now, I was in my early 30's at the time and he was in his late 60's, but I didn't care! And, seriously, have you noticed how fast some 60-year-olds are?

Runners are probably one of the only groups of people who get excited about getting older. That means a new age group. When you turn 40, you become a "Masters Runner". Sounds impressive, doesn't it! Also, each new age group is a new opportunity to set personal records. And, the longer you hang around, the fewer runners in your age group!

I do need to tell you one more age group award story. We went to a race in the middle of farm country here in Virginia. The race was a 10K race held the Saturday before Thanksgiving. Age group winners got.....yep, you're right......a turkey! I was even happier to win my age group that year – I didn't have to buy the main course for Thanksgiving dinner!

Another thing about races is the t-shirts that you collect. Most all races give a t-shirt when you sign up. After so many years and races, the t-shirts start to accumulate. There are companies out there that will take your race shirts and make plaques or quilts with them. A friend of mine had some of his made into a quilt. I have to admit – it's pretty cool!

Some races put a lot of thought into their shirts and some well.......let's just say that there are some in the drawer that won't come out again! The local running club here actually had an ugly race shirt contest one year at our Christmas Party. There are definitely some ugly ones out there.

But, there are some that I treasure! Most of my marathon shirts are pretty great – and I love my Disney World Marathon ones. Another race that has some nice shirts is the Rock and Roll Marathon and Half-marathon series races. Those are ones that I will wear around a lot.

Nowadays, there are races that will give you moisture-wicking shirts that you can wear to run in. These are great and I also love the races that will give you race jackets and hats. It's a lot more than just cotton t-shirts.

My race shirts are my badges of honor. I love wearing them around!

Chapter 7 - What??? I Won???

This is a story that will just prove that you never know what will happen when you enter a race.

Several years ago, I entered a 10K race about an hour from my home. It was one of those races where there was a 5K and a 10K. Whenever you can enter for more than one race, I always go for the longer race. This goes back to my not being fast – but having endurance.

This was a real nice race along some back country roads. It was one of those races where everyone started and then the shorter race peeled off onto another road. But, it wasn't an out and back – so you really didn't know who was in what race or who was still ahead of you.

As I was coming up to the finish line, I took a look at my watch. It was going to be a decent time for me. Not my fastest 10K, but a pretty good time. When I crossed the finish line, I kept hearing, "Congratulations!", "Way to go!". I thought how nice it was the way they congratulated everyone when they finished.

Then, I found out why. I had actually won for overall female for the 10K! Me – win a race? Never in my wildest dreams – but here I was! I got a nice Silver Bowl for winning that I still have. And, my picture in the paper! Hearing my name as the overall female winner during the awards was feeling that I'll never forget.

Now, I'm not sure how many females actually ran in the 10K part of the race that day. But, you know what? I don't care. I won – and I've got the bowl and newspaper clipping to prove it!

Chapter 8 – My First Marathon

As with every runner, I decided that I wanted to run a marathon. In my mind, that was just the ultimate. Running a marathon would show my dedication to my sport and would show that I had the dedication and motivation to do the training involved.

So, training began. I bought the book, *The Competitive Runner's Handbook* by Bob Glover and followed the marathon training schedule for novices religiously. Whatever the book said – I did most of the time. (But, the streaker that I am – rest days in the schedule meant 2 miles to me).

The marathon that I decided to do for my first was the Marine Corps Marathon in Washington, D.C. It's a great race for many reasons and a wonderful race for first time marathoners. So, a few days before the race, off to Washington we went.

There was a group of us that traveled up to Washington together. I think there were 3 cars of us. Well, one of the runners definitely took the "hydrate a few days before the race" a little too seriously. I didn't think we'd ever get to D.C. Every rest area we passed, we had to stop for him. I wish I had counted how many times we stopped that day. I think someone finally hid his water and Gatorade bottles!

When we got to Washington, we did the usual pre-race things. Went to the expo, picked up my race packet, etc. The group that I traveled to D.C. with went to dinner at a wonderful Italian restaurant for our pre-race pasta meal. Then, it was finally here. Race day! And, it was an absolutely beautiful day! Sunny and 55 degrees! A perfect November morning!

As anyone running their first marathon should, my goal for the race was strictly to finish. I had run up to 22 miles in training, but I had read enough to know that those last few miles can be pretty unpredictable.

I ran the marathon just as I read about in my training book. I started out fairly slowly to warm up and then just let the miles go by. This course is absolutely wonderful. It winds through most of the monuments and you can get lost in thought as you pass by all that history.

Before I knew it, I was at mile 20. Really? Already? It really didn't feel that bad at all – I know, relatively speaking! The last 6 miles were a little tougher, but I really did feel good. And, I had the confidence that I had trained hard and correctly for the distance.

The Marine Corps Marathon finishes at the Marine Corps War Memorial. It is just a great feeling when you round the last corner and there you are! Such a rush of emotion! A young man about 25 or so finished right in front of me. I'll never forget that finish. His dad was right there and they both hugged each other and burst into tears.

I was a little teary-eyed myself. It was a great feeling to accomplish such a goal. And, I had worked hard and had finished strong – breaking 4 hours for my first marathon!

And, as an extra special moment, not only was my wonderful hubby there at the finish line – but my parents had surprised me and traveled over 4 hours to see me finish! It was a special day all around! One that I'll never forget!

Chapter 9 - "Runner's World" Days

Now, I've never been featured in Runner's World Magazine, and probably never will be. "Runner's World" Days refers to days that I've run, that warrant a picture in Runner's World. We declared those days as such many years ago – yes, during one of those days.

The first one that I can remember is when I still lived in my hometown. I went out for a 10-miler, weather looked good, no big deal. But then, about 5 miles into my run, the sky started to cloud up a little. Still alright, and then, at about 7, the sky got mad!

The most horrendous thunderstorm that I've ever been outside in started. Horrendous rains and thunder and lightning. Here's the deal, I don't do thunderstorms very well when I'm inside let alone when I'm out in it and being a human lightning rod!

About a mile from home, an extremely loud and close clap of thunder shook me to the core. I came up on a Church. What a better and safer place to be than a Church, right? So, dripping wet and scared to death, I stood right there on their steps under an awning until the thunder and lightning subsided.

Now, I know that I was only a short distance from home, but I definitely felt better being right there on those Church steps!

Then, there were the days when I lived there in the winter time. One winter was unusually brutal. For several days, it below 0 and one day it was about -20 when I went running. My Gore-Tex suit was definitely my best friend those days.

On those days (and we won't even go into wind chill added), I'd have on 2 or 3 layers of shirts under my Gore-Tex jacket. Then, I'd have tights on under my pants. A toboggan under the hood and then a mask over my mouth and nose. I'm sure I was a sight. No speed work on those days! Bob always laughed at me when I'd come in with icy eyelashes.

Then, there was the ice. I actually bought the gear that you hook onto your running shoes that have spikes in them to give you traction on the ice. They're really pretty cool if you live in areas where you have to deal with icy roads.

Some runners like running in the colder weather – but on really cold days like that now – it's the treadmill for me!

Then, there was the day of my hurricane run. I was in Virginia Beach for a half-marathon Labor Day week-end several years ago. A hurricane was coming up the coast - but not expected to be a threat to the area. Well, Friday evening and Saturday morning - we got a part of it!

We definitely got a lot of wind and rain. It was so bad that the concerts that were scheduled for Friday night were canceled. But, Saturday morning, I had to get out for my run. A little hurricane isn't going to stop the streak.

Luckily, I had seen the weather forecast before I left home and had my rain gear with me. Out the door and down the boardwalk I went. Good thing that it was a short and easy run before the race the next day. I managed to get a couple of miles in. The wind was so strong that at many times I was running - but not moving forward.

And, just to let you know - I wasn't the only one out there that day. There were a bunch of us crazies!

The next morning, for race day, was absolutely beautiful! You'd never believe that it was so bad just the day before.

Now, I'm not saying that you should go out and run in a hurricane. I knew that it was fairly safe when I ran in the one I did. It wasn't the dangerous part of the storm – and it was growing weaker. I may be a streaker – but not stupid! But, I do have a pretty cool story from it. Not everyone can say that they've run in a hurricane!

Chapter 10 – Funny Running Stories

Every runner has stories – some they can share – and probably some that they can't! But I've had my share of funny stories, also.

My favorite running story happened many years ago, when I still lived in the town I grew up in. I ran the same 5 mile route every morning early before I got ready to go to work. And, every morning Monday through Friday, I saw the same mail truck. Not a delivery truck, but the larger box trucks that take mail from one post office to another.

Every morning, we'd pass each other. I'd smile and wave. He'd honk his horn and wave. One year on Christmas Eve, I could see him coming in the distance. (I knew it was him, at 5:30 on this road back then, there wasn't a lot of traffic.). As he got closer to me, he slowed down and pulled over to the side of the road.

He actually got out and gave me a 5 pound box of candy for Christmas! How sweet was that? I thanked him SO much, he got back in his truck and headed on up the road. Luckily, I was only about 1 ½ miles from home, so it was just a little weight workout carrying my candy home.

It was just one of those things that probably would never happen again. It was a great Christmas present and gave me a running memory that I'll never forget.

Another story involves my husband. We had a date schedule for a Sunday evening after I had some friends from college visit for the week-end. (I had graduated a semester early – so it was a nice visit.) And, it was actually our first date. He had asked me out 2 other times, but this was the first time that we were scheduled to go out. (Long story for another time!).

Late Sunday afternoon, after my friends left, I headed out for my run. I had plenty of time before Bob was picking me up for our movie date. As I was heading home, he stopped and asked if I wanted to eat before we went to the movies. Of course I said yes, and he said that he would pick me up at a certain time.

Bob drove off and then I looked at my watch. I had an hour to finish my run (about a mile from home) and get cleaned up for our date. That was probably one of the fastest miles that I've ever run. But, I made it and we had a great time!

Rocky is involved in another story. Well, actually the Rocky statue in Philadelphia! I was in Philly for a business conference. 2 of the people with us were also runners. Planning our run one morning, we decided that it just wouldn't be right to run there without doing the "Rocky steps". So, we asked directions at the front desk and we were off.

We made our way around the streets of Philadelphia and suddenly there it was! The museum with the Rocky Statue. So, up the steps we went. And, being the pure running geeks that we are, once we got to the top - we did the jumping up and down with our arms in the air – just like Rocky. And, of course, we were humming the Rocky Theme!

There are many crazy stories from my years of running, but those are 3 of my favorites!

Chapter 11 – Running Through Sickness

I have been blessed with good health – which I do attribute to my running – and to running everyday. I rarely get a cold – and when I do, it doesn't last very long at all. I feel that running has kept me healthier – and keeps everything internally working in good order.

However, there have been a few times when I've not felt the greatest. But, I ran through it. Most of the time thanks to my treadmill. If you're feeling puny, best to have something to hang onto (the side rails) if you need to. Here are a few of those stories.

The first time that I can remember being really sick was in the mid-1990's. I came down with a case of the shingles. The worst that I have ever felt – and have never felt as bad since. But, I wasn't going to end the streak. Down to the treadmill I went everyday – I really looked too bad to go outside.

I made myself run a mile everyday. And, believe it or not, I was over the shingles in one week. Nobody could believe that I was better that quickly. I firmly believe that running helped me heal. Sweating out the nastiness was the best thing I could have done.

There were a couple of days when I really didn't know if I would make it or not. But, I'm glad I did. I got better quicker – and, most importantly, the streak continued!

The next time was really not a sickness, but a procedure that I needed to have done. I was at the age where my doctor wanted me to have a colonoscopy. So, he sent me to the doctor who would be doing it for a consultation and explanation of everything.

He got to the morning of. I asked him if I could run that morning. He looked at me quizzically, so I explained everything to him. I told him about my streak, how long that it was and how important it was to me not to miss a day of running.

The doctor kind of laughed, but told me it was OK to do a short run – and not to overdo it. I promised him 1 mile only – and thanked him for understanding. So, the morning of, I got my run in early before I headed to the hospital.

The only other time was just this past year. My husband and I both had some kind of bug that really hit us hard. We didn't want to eat and it totally zapped our energy. We stayed in bed most of a week and a half.

The first day, it got to be late afternoon before I could get the strength to get out of bed, dressed and downstairs to the treadmill. I was almost crying. But, down I went and got my run done. Wasn't pretty, definitely wasn't fast – but it was done. The rest of the week went much better after that.

Running through sicknesses is not for everybody. But, I know that it helps me to feel better quicker. I'm just thankful that I have my treadmill for those days – and that my husband understands!

Chapter 12 – My Favorite Races

I'm going to break this up into 2 parts. First of all, I'm going to talk about my favorite road race period. Then, I'm going to fill you in on my 3 favorite marathons.

My Favorite Road Race

My favorite race is one that I've run for many years. I always make sure that it's on my racing schedule every year. The Rock and Roll Half-Marathon in Virginia Beach is absolutely fantastic! It's run the Sunday of Labor Day week-end during the American Music Festival and Bob and I have really come to look forward to this week-end every year. It's just nice to enjoy a week-end on the beach. Good food, sunshine, beach - we make this a relaxing time together!

There are stages for the bands set up at several areas of the beach - if you plan it right, you can sit on your balcony and listen to the bands in the evenings throughout the week-end. In the past few years, we've listened to Steve Miller Band, Starship, Heart and many more - yes I do love 70's and 80's music. There are other types of music at the other stages. After the bands finish at night, there are fireworks over the ocean.

The race itself is great! 13 miles around Virginia Beach and some of it is run on the boardwalk. It's great! Also, along the race route are local bands set up playing that really gets you energized! As you run through the neighborhoods, there are people cheering - they even have contests for the best cheering crowds!

If you're looking for a fun run destination week-end, you just can't beat the Rock and Roll Half-Marathon in Virginia Beach!

My 3 Favorite Marathons

Many marathons are great for a destination race.
Here are my 3 favorite full marathons.

1. Disney Marathon - I've run this marathon 3
times. I love this race -   even with the 6 a.m. start!
You know what kind of a show Disney puts on - so
imagine what they can do to a marathon.

Mickey and Minnie Mouse start you on your way
with fireworks in the background. Then you run
through all the theme parks and finish up at Epcot.
There are fans and "characters" all along the route.
A nicely done race. And, it's run in Florida in
January - important in my book!

2. A1A Marathon – This is another race that I've
run several times. What a great run! If you're not
familiar with Florida, A1A is a route that goes along
the coast. It's another early start - but watching the
sunrise over the ocean is always breathtaking. The
finish (by the way the race is in Fort Lauderdale) is

in a park along the beach where they always have a super sand sculpture. Oh, yeah, it's in Florida in February.

3. Marine Corps Marathon - not a race in Florida in the winter, but just a super race that I've run multiple times. It's a great marathon for first-timers. I love Washington, D.C. and the history there. This race is run around the city and all the monuments. The support along this course is second to none - Marines are at all the aid stations with whatever you may need. This race is always run in late October or early November.

I've run many marathons, but these are 3 of my favorites. If you're going to run 26.2 miles, you may as well have some fun and see some sights along the way!

Chapter 13 – DNF Is Not In My Vocabulary

DNF means "did not finish". That is something that no runner wants to see beside their name in race results. Now, things can happen to cause you not to finish – especially during a marathon. If not properly trained, you can run out of steam, muscle cramps if you don't keep hydrated, etc. But, most runners, will do anything to finish, even if they have to crawl across the finish line.

I'm one of those runners. Now, I've been blessed and lucky that I've never had anything too extreme happen to cause me to not finish. But, a few years ago, I ran a marathon that definitely tested my resolve.

The race was the Shamrock Marathon in Virginia Beach. About halfway into the race, I fell. To this day, I don't know what happened, but down I went.

And I don't know about you, but I never fall gracefully. I'm sure it was a sight to see.

Anyway, I fell mostly on one knee. I looked down, saw a little blood, but kept on going. Now, remember, this is 13 miles into 26. I still had a long way to go.

At first, my body was a little stiff from the fall, but after a few miles, it let up some. I had almost forgotten about the bloody knee until the turnaround point in a park. A friend I knew saw me and asked me what happened – as he was pointing to my knee. There was a stream of dried blood that was running down my leg. Oh, well, I'm sure it looked worse than it was.

Around 20 miles, my knee and leg that I fell on started to get sore again. But, I was determined to finish. My motto was (and still is): "I've never DNF'd, and I'm not going to now". A couple of times, I walked through the water stop to take a little rest – and to make sure that I took in all the water I could

– hydration had to help, right? Anyway, I finished. That is one finisher's medal that I am really proud of.

Chapter 14 – My Running Heroes

There are two runners that were at their prime in the 70's that will always be my running heroes. I've added a few others since I first started running – they all inspire me to be out there every day.

Bill Rodgers was in his prime when I first started running in the 70's. He won the Boston and New York Marathon numerous times and I feel that he is one of the greatest runners of all time! His 2:09:27 winning time in the 1979 Boston Marathon was an American Record at the time, and remains his PR.

I love his easy going style. And, he is so accessible to his fans - not like other elite athletes. Bill is always willing to talk to anyone, give autographs, stand for pictures, etc. I know this for a fact - I have several racing bibs with his name autographed on them. I actually met him and had my picture taken with him one year at the Charleston Distance Race. It's something that I'll always treasure!

Bill and his brother also opened a running center in Boston and he had a line of running clothes. I haven't worn them in years - they're a little worn - but I still have a couple of Gore-Tex running suits that are from his line. I just can't seem to part with them!

Now, that he's older (like the rest of us), he's still out there running races. He'll probably never win a major race again - but he's still out there. Running for the pure enjoyment of it. I can SO relate to that.

The second running hero of mine is who I feel is the greatest women's runner of all time - Grete Waitz!

Grete was a long-distance runner from Norway. She was also at her prime around the time that I started running. I wanted to be just like her - tall, slender - and I did wear my hair in pig-tails like hers at times!

The first year that she ran the New York marathon, she not only won it - but took 2 minutes off the women's world record. She went on to win New York 9 times!

Grete was not only a great marathon runner - she ran other distances as well. I saw her one year at the Charleston Distance Run - a 15-miler in Charleston, West Virginia. It was absolutely great to see her run in person. She did, however, finish her 15 miles while I was at the 10-mile mark!

Grete started running in her home country of Norway in a time when women, as runners, were really not taken seriously. In 1975, she was one of the first women to run the 3000 meters in competitive races. She broke the world record twice that year in that distance and for the first time realized that she was part of a revolution that tried to attain equality for female athletes.

In April of 2011, Grete lost her long-running battle with cancer. She will be missed!

In the last few years, I developed a few more running heroes.

Jeff Galloway is one of my newer heroes – even though I've been reading his books for years. He is another runner who has been out on the roads for many years.

One of his books , Galloway's Book On Running is probably one of the first running books I ever read. It's the Bible for most runners.

Jeff was an Olympic runner in the 70's and is still out there running. He was the first winner of the Peachtree Road Race in Atlanta and after that was instrumental in making it the wonderful, international race it is today.

Jeff has a passion for helping runners get started running and keep on running through their life. (I can totally relate to that!). He now coaches many runners to their first races and first marathons with his run/walk program.

And, I love his book on Running Until You're 100. That's how I feel – and he gives great tips for staying with your running program.

Dean Karnazes is another one of my new heroes. I love the things that he's accomplished. The running of 50 marathons in 50 days and running across the United States are just two of his accomplishments. He does these runs to promote charities. I would love to do some terrific feats like he has! His books are wonderful to read and great inspiration!

I think about doing ultra runs (races of more than a marathon) from time to time. I do plan on doing one some day. Dean is the person that I get inspiration from.

John Bingham is another one of my newer heroes. He is known as The Penguin and writes The Penguin Chronicles. I feel a special kinship with him – especially as I keep running as I get older. John, also was not an athlete in high school and started running later. His famous quote is "The miracle isn't that I finished. The miracle is that I had the courage to start."

That's exactly how I feel. It doesn't matter how fast you run – it's just the fact that you're out there that does.

Well, those are my heroes. Each of them motivates me a little each day. Having someone to look up to is important!

Chapter 15 – Bodily Functions and Running

Now, this is an area that all long-distance runners deal with – whether they want to admit it or not. What to do if you need to relieve yourself during your run or race. Running can make a person be not so modest.

During long runs, sometimes you just can't find a convenience store or place to go. So, you look for bushes that are big enough to hide you from the road. Now, you may think this is wrong – but if you've ever been out there for a 2+ hour run, you're a mile or so from the closest place with "facilities" - trust me, you do what you need to do!

It also happens at races. Now, if you've ever been to a major race – you know that there are port-a-potties around the starting line. But, you also know that if you wait too long, you risk not starting on time. Now, I always plan to come out of one and get right back in line, so I don't worry about it.

Others are not so lucky. There are many races where you'll see people peeling off during the first mile when you get to the first grove of trees or even a wall. It's actually kind of comical to watch. Longer races have port-a-potties along the course, but usually farther in. So, they take care of things then and there.

Now, I try to never stop during a race. I watch what I eat the morning of the race and watch my water intake the ½ hour before. But, I have stopped a time or two when I needed to. 26.2 miles is a long way.

There are some races that begin at a school or other building. Usually, you are fighting a long line because of limited bathrooms. And, we all know that the ladies' line is always longer than the men's line. No problem. I have no issues with going into a men's room if it's empty. You just have someone as a look-out and then you do the same for them. Like I said, you do what you've got to do!

During a race there are two things you have to watch out for – nose blowers and spitters. I don't have any problem with this myself, but I do have some running friends that do. When they need to blow their nose, they put their finger on one nostril and blow out the other. Seriously, would they do this in the real world? Then there are the spitters. People who would never think about spitting in public have absolutely no problem with doing it in a race.

Just remember when you are in the middle of a race – if you see someone in front of you slightly turn their head – Be Aware!

Chapter 16 – Preventing Injuries

I've been lucky in the fact that I've never had a serious injury. I listen to my body and cut back on days that I'm not quite up to par. But, it's a runner's biggest fear. Getting injured and not being able to run. Here are some ways to prevent running injuries.

1. Commit yourself to a warm-up. The general rule in any type of workout: Warm-up before you go. Doing so gives you a chance to prepare your body for the oncoming work and prevents the likelihood of injuries. Before a run, loosen up your legs, walk for some minutes, then do some stretching. Similarly, cooling down at the end of the run is important to reduce muscle pain. Do this by closing your workout with brisk walking or slow running. Then, do stretches.

Personally, I don't like to stretch before I go out. I just start my run slowly for the first 1/2 mile or so until I get warmed up.

2. Avoid overtraining. The surest way to incur injuries is to overtrain and overwork your body. Sadly, many runners, in an attempt to increase their mileage and intensity just too soon, push their body beyond its capability and so put their selves at a great risk of injury. Two things you need to remember. One, weekly mileage increase shouldn't be more than 10%. Two, speed buildup is a gradual process. Next time you feel like going farther and faster, ask if your body is capable of the demands, then let sound judgment overtake you.

3. Take some breaks. This is especially important if you feel soreness in your muscles or are overly tired. A day or two of missed run is better than subjecting your already fatigued body to a possibility of injury. Listen to your body well and

take note of pain, or any other hint, that tries to communicate it is not up for the challenge.

4. Use good shoes. You know you need to replace your shoes when they have reached around 300 to 400 miles. By then, their shock absorption has degraded and their soles have worn-out, leaving them unsafe for running.

5. Keep from concrete surfaces. Not only are they hard, they also are not a very good shock absorber. Instead, run on dirt or grass trails, or somewhere there is a soft surface. This will put less pressure on your legs.

6. Do cross-training activities. The purpose of cross-training is to develop and strengthen your running muscles through other physical means such as swimming, biking, and hiking. It is best to incorporate cross-training activities in your running

program at least once a week. Remember, however, that cross-training activities are supposed to improve your stamina and not to stress your body out and leave you with less energy for running.

7. Observe rehabilitation measures should you suspect any injury. Doing so will prevent injury complications and speed up the recovery process. You can do a massage and cold therapy to ease a minor injury. For more serious cases, consult with a doctor immediately.

As I always say, listen to your body. If it says it needs a rest day, take the day off or just run a slow and easy run that day. It's worked for me and I'm sure it will work for you.

Chapter 17 – Running and Nutrition

Like a car, a runner who wants to operate at his most optimum potential needs his particular set of fuels. He needs the right combination of carbohydrates, proteins and fats - the correct fuel for runners.

Each of these food groups has a specific function to fulfill in the body. Getting the right amount and mix of these important nutrients is important.

Carbohydrates

The primary fuel for exercising muscles and for high-intensity exercises are carbohydrates. The athlete's body needs around 50 to 65% carbohydrates in his food intake to support training.

Lacking enough carbohydrates causes the body to under-perform and cannot burn fats as effectively as it should during workouts. It should be the staple of your diet before, during and after each exercise, including intervals throughout the day.

Carbohydrates are found in such food as whole grain breads, pasta, brown rice, oatmeal, fruits, vegetables, potatoes, corn, beans, and low-fat dairy products.

Proteins

Proteins are important because they build and repair muscles, ligaments, and tendons –all essentials in becoming a strong athlete.

You can get your proteins from such sources as egg whites, poultry (with the skin), fish, ground turkey or chicken breast, lean ground beef, game meat, nuts, tofu and soy milk and low-fat dairy products.

Proteins are important to take in after a hard race or workout. This is because proteins help the body repair itself after strenuous activities.

Fats

The last food group, fat, helps sustain prolonged exercises at lower intensities. Our bodies have enough stored fat to fuel prolonged exercise. However, fat is difficult to use for quick energy. This is why carbohydrates are the choice fuel during most exercises.

Athletes need about 20 to 30% of calories from fats. Healthy sources of fats include fatty fish (salmon for omega 3 fatty acids), nuts and natural peanut butter, avocado, olive oil, and canola oil.

Correct balance

For an athlete, achieving the right balance of these three all-important food groups is the step to fulfill your potential. Your day-to-day diet has to be adjusted accordingly to support your training.

As always, listening to your body is the most important thing you can do. If you're continually feeling draggy, maybe you need to take a look at your diet.

Chapter 18 – Why You Should Be A Runner

Running is a great all-around activity. Some runners get started simply as a means to losing a few excess pounds. Others have started running for the over-all sense of well-being it gives them. I feel that there are 11 basic reasons to start (or keep) running.

1. Weight loss is a great by-product. Running is one of the best calorie burners there is. The amount of calories you burn depends on how much you weigh, the terrain that you are running on and the weather conditions. For instance, you'll work harder running into the wind and running uphill. Thus, burning more calories.

More calories are burned running than by aerobics or working out on an exercise bike. And, the more you weigh, the more calories you'll burn. Another plus, once you build muscle, you will burn off calories more quickly – muscle requires more energy.

2. Psychological benefits. Runners seem to be less stressed and handle things better than non-runners. They also seem to develop a more focused mind. I know that I always do my best thinking – and come up with my best ideas – while I'm out on my run.

Runners seem to be less depressed. They seem to be able to heal mentally and are more aware of themselves. I know that running is my therapy!

3. Running gives you more energy. I know that there are those of you that may say that's crazy. You use so much energy to run – how can it give you more? It does. Regular exercise has been shown to increase energy levels. I'm an early morning runner and I know that running gives me energy throughout my whole day.

4. Running is absolutely free! You don't need to join a gym, you don't need to pay monthly fees, you don't need to buy fancy equipment - just lace up your shoes and head out the door!

5. Running keeps you young. Another one that I don't know the physical, inner medical workings behind this - but I know I feel many years younger than I am. Running seems to give you a glow and keeps everything toned up.

6. Running is a great stress reliever! If you had a bad day, or have something going on in your life - lace up your shoes and go head out the door. It will really clear your mind - and is much cheaper than a therapist!

7. It is your "me" time. Being an only child, I enjoy a little time to myself. If you have a busy lifestyle, it's not always easy to do....job....children....spouse. But, running will get you that sanity time that you need!

8. Think through things. Running is great for sorting through things that you may be dealing with. I've reasoned through many problems, come up with great ideas - you'll be surprised how many things you'll solve during your runs.

9. It gets you outside. I work from home - so running is my time to get out and enjoy the outdoors. Even if you work in an office - getting out in the fresh air is important. And that's good for everyone!

10. Help a charity. Once you get started running, you may want to enter a race to earn money for a charity. There are so many races and groups that raise money from road races. It's an easy way to help out others.

11. Medical benefits. Runners have been

shown to have lower blood pressure, better cholesterol levels, etc. Running just keeps you healthy inside and out!

Chapter 19 – Psychological Benefits Of Running

We all know that running is great for keeping your physical body in shape. But, did you know that it can also keep you in good mental health?

1. Running helps to reduce stress and anxiety. Runners are known to be less stressed and are more able to deal with their daily stressors effectively. This is attributed to the fact that running refreshes their thoughts, keeps their minds off worries, and gives them ample and undistracted time to think, reflect, and concentrate. In addition, according to some reports, running is more efficient in addressing anxieties better than medications.

2. Running enhances your moods. When running, the body produces a substance called endorphin (endogenous morphine) that creates a different sense of euphoria. This state of euphoria is called

runner's high basically because after running, individuals are in a good mood, are happier, and indescribably feel better. Runner's high is also believed to be responsible for the runners' seeming "addiction" to running: Because they are always intensely post-euphoric, runners keep running every chance they get.

3. Runners experience improved confidence. The sense of achievement after finishing a run or completing a target distance boosts the runners' confidence. This is especially true of people who are naturally competitive - they regularly sign up for marathons and other running events. Improved confidence also comes to people who have noticeably lost weight and achieved more toned and firmer muscles through running.

4. Any addictions you may have can be fought by running. Running is conceived to be a natural tranquilizer, which is why therapists recommend it to those who are battling with their addiction. Many

successful stories have been documented, saying that recovering patients use the time they would otherwise spend to satisfy their addiction in running. Through running, patients also become mentally stronger to resist the urge of alcohol, drugs, or anything they feel addicted to.

5. Running will help you to achieve mental alertness and focus. Because running keeps the mind on the "now," the mind is trained to focus and concentrate. Running also relieves mental fatigue, sharpens memory, and improves overall mental stamina. Runners, in effect, are found to have better problem-solving skills and are more mentally alert than before.

6. Running is found successful in treating clinical depression. The act of running, according to therapists, serves as a psychotherapy, which gives the patients their own space to heal and connect with their selves better. They also say it is a good distraction from all depressing things. Other than

depression, physicians also find running an effective therapy for people with other types of psychological disorders.

7. The coordination of mind and body is improved with regular running. Whether running on a flat, paved surface or on an uneven trail, the mind is trained to harmoniously work with the body to prevent stumbling and tripping over. Like the other psychological benefits of running, better mind-body coordination is important in daily activities.

I absolutely love the fact that my running is also helping my mind to stay sharp!

Chapter 20 – Dressing for Different Types of Weather

As a runner, it would be wonderful if the weather was always perfect. But, we all know that is certainly not the case. We have to deal with hot weather running and cold weather running. And, then there's wind and rain.

So, during all those years that I've been running, I've pretty much run in all types of weather. Here are some tips for running during those "not so perfect" days.

Winter Running

Winter running doesn't have to be miserable. In fact, it can be enjoyable if you are wearing the proper running apparel. An important thing to remember is that you'll feel better during your run if you are wearing comfortable clothes. Whether you are a fairly new runner running a mile or a seasoned runner training for longer distances, the clothes you're wearing can make a difference. And, it's especially important to have proper clothes for winter running.

 Runners should wear clothing that is not only comfortable, but "runner friendly". What I mean by that is that you should wear apparel made with moisture-wicking fabrics. This fabric will "wick" away the moisture from your body as you sweat and keep you dry. This is important in both cold weather and warmer weather. If you wear shirts that don't do this - as you sweat, the sweat stays against your body, you stay wet, cold and pretty miserable.

Cotton is the one fabric that you want to stay away from. Cotton will absorb your body heat, your moisture as your sweat and will cling to your body. This makes your run pretty miserable no matter what time of year it is. Most runners that have been running for years can attest to this. We've all been out there in our cotton t-shirts before better material became available.

Layering your clothing is the best way to stay comfortable when you are running in colder weather. Multiple layers will keep you drier than one heavy piece of apparel. The different layers will keep you warm while wicking moisture away from your body. How many layers you wear depends on a couple of factors - how cold the climate is your running in, is it raining and how warm you like to be when you run.

Another good thing to remember is that you should dress as if it is 10 degrees warmer than it actually is outside. The extra 10 degrees accounts for your body heat.

Your base layer is the most important. This layer needs to move moisture away from you so that you won't get chilled. This is the layer where you definitely want a technical shirt - such as CoolMax. For some runners, this layer could be a singlet or for others a long sleeve shirt.

A shirt with a zipper that is a great next layer - especially if you are using 2 layers. If it gets a little warmer, you can partially unzip and allow some ventilation. If it turns cooler on you or the wind starts to pick up - you can zip it all the way up.

When the weather is really cold or if it's raining/snowing, you need some sort of jacket. You can find jackets now that are wind-resistant and water resistant. When you are looking at jackets, make sure to look to see if they are venting in the back (and sometimes under the arms). This will allow the ventilation that you need so that your layers don't get "heavy" as you sweat.

You also want to remember your hands and feet. Be sure to wear gloves and a hat or band over your ears on those super cold days. Also, If it's raining, I like to wear a cap that is rain-resistant. This keeps the rain from getting in my eyes.

Running in the winter can be a lot of fun if you make sure you are properly prepared for it. Just remember, you want to stay comfortable, warm and dry!

Summer Running

I love when the weather gets warmer and the running shorts out of the drawer! But, with the warmer weather, there are some things that you need to be aware of for your running. Here are some tips for how to dress for your runs.

The cotton tee shirts that you receive at races are great - and pretty neat to wear around - but you don't want to wear them during your runs. Cotton will hold your sweat and not dry quickly. Even though they cost a little more - you really want to buy technical material shirts such as CoolMax. These materials will wick the moisture away from your skin - and will cause a cooling effect as you run. Once you wear them, especially on a longer run, you'll definitely feel the difference.

And, while we're talking about cotton, you don't want to wear 100% cotton socks. Your feet sweat a lot during runs and the same as shirts - it will hold in the moisture. Once cotton gets wet - it stays wet. This can lead to blisters. Make sure you are wearing some sort of moisture-wicking socks.

Break out those shades! A nice pair of running sunglasses will protect your eyes and help with the glare. Also, if you are running longer distances in the bright sunshine, squinting for a long period of time can cause headaches. Make sure they fit you well. There is nothing more annoying than sunglasses bobbing up and down on your nose.

Also, I like to wear a cap. This will also help with the glare and shade your face.

I like to wear bright colors anyway, but during the summer it is especially important. Light colored clothing will reflect the light from the sun while dark colors will absorb it. Also, make sure your clothing is loose-fitting. Tight-fitting clothing can keep your body from breathing as it should to cool down naturally.

And, on a side note - make sure you stay hydrated. Drink before you head out on your run. Also, if you are running long - plan on water stops along your route. I always carry a gold dollar coin with me for stopping at a convenience store for water. (I hate to give someone a soggy dollar bill).

Personally, I love running during the summer weather! You just have to make sure you are doing it safely and dressing correctly!

Running In The Wind

OK, I'll be the first one to admit it - I hate running in the wind. Somehow, it's alright if I'm running along the beach - but that's another story. But, running on windy days is something that we all have to learn to cope with. Here are some tips for running in the wind.

1. Plan your run so that you start out heading out facing into the wind. This gives you a little extra work-out with the resistance heading out. Doing this will also help you on the way back. You'll be a little tired from the extra energy exerted - so the wind will help push you on your way back.

2. Lean into the wind. If you lean into the wind - it will help deflect it a little. Think car racing. If you're not running totally upright, you'll have some resistance against the wind.

3. Relax your shoulders. Many runners want to run tense up and lift their shoulders when running during windy days. Keeping your shoulders relaxed will help keep you from having muscle soreness in your neck and shoulders after your run.

4. Remember that your pace will be slower with the wind in your face. But, then, you'll be faster once you turn around! Studies show that your pace can increase by about 5% with the wind at your back, but when you are running into the wind your pace can decrease by about 8%. This was done at 10 mph winds - so imagine the workout you're getting at 25 mph winds! Just know that it's OK if you're running slower - but remember you may be getting a better workout with the extra resistance.

5. Drink your water. On windy days - the wind will dry the sweat from you. Remember that sweat on your skin in a good thing for cooling your body. So, be sure you're keeping up with your water intake.

6. Dress for the wind. This is especially true if you are running in a cold wind. Make sure that you are dressing in layers - you need to protect yourself from wind chill. Your top layer should be a kind of technical, wind-resistant material to help with this.

Also, remember to wear lip balm to help keep moisture in your lips. Trust me, dry and cracked lips are not fun. I always keep a tube in my pocket. If you're on the road for awhile, it will wear off - plus if you stop for water, you need to reapply your lip balm.

7. Try to run in the early morning if you know it's going to be a windy day. This helps me SO much. It seems that around dawn, the winds settle down. If it's been windy all night - they let up for a little bit. If it's going to be a windy day - they usually don't kick up until later in the morning.

Running in the wind doesn't have to be all that bad. Just follow the above tips and I'm sure you'll be fine!

There are some tips for running in many types of weather. They've worked for me – and I'm sure that they will work for you!

Chapter 21 – Just Be Safe

Running is great – but you also need to take precautions. Be smart and be safe!

The Importance of Wearing ID When You Run

Most runners, myself included, think that they are pretty much invincible while they are out on the run. They think that nothing can happen to them and have a false sense of security all the time.

The truth is - there are many things that a runner needs to be aware of. There are always the anticipated problems - heavy traffic areas, icy roads, excessive heat, etc. However, there are some unforeseen dangers that can happen, especially if you run alone - as I do.

Unexpected weather conditions, medical conditions, wild animals or even attacks by people. OK, I don't mean to scare you from going out alone - but you need to be aware that things can happen. In over 35 years of running, nothing has ever happened to me out on the roads by myself, but I know that they can.

If you are training for a longer race - you may be out on the roads for 2-4 hours. Many things can happen during that much time out. So, it's important to be prepared. And, you need to keep in mind that you may not be able to give someone the information that they need to help you.

The personal identification that you carry should include: your name, your emergency contact(s), their phone number (depending on what time you usually run - you may include their work number, cell, etc), any medical conditions you have, any allergies you have and possibly your primary care physician. On my ID is my name, our home phone number, my husband's name and his cell phone number and our address.

My husband feels so much better with the knowledge that I have identification on me. He worries when I'm out for over an hour - and I'm sure your loved ones do, too!

I got my personal identifications from Road ID. I love it! I believe in simplicity when I run and didn't want something bulky or something that I had to wear. The first one that I got velcros onto my shoe - so I don't even know it's there. It's great.

Then, Road ID came out with a great bracelet. It's lightweight and comes in many colors. Mine is a pretty pink!

If you run longer runs, having this identification on you is important. And, it gives your loved ones peace of mind!

Treadmills Are OK

There are many runners that I know that think that "treadmill" is a dirty word. And, I'll admit, I used to be one of those runners. But, not for many years now. Now, there are days when my treadmill is my best friend! I've learned to accept – and appreciate treadmill running!

There was a time when I would run in any kind of weather. I've run in temperatures of 20 below, blizzards, hurricanes, thunderstorms, etc. It never fazed me. Many times, my hubby would laugh at me when I came in from a winter run with my eyelashes frozen. But, I had to run – it didn't matter what the weather was. And, go to a gym and run on a treadmill – never!

Well, for several years, my husband used to travel during the week. He worried about me during the winter. He was afraid of me running when it was icy outside. So, he talked me into buying a treadmill. And, basically just to pacify him, I did.

Then, a bad storm hit. It was snowy, icy and about 0 degrees. I didn't get off work until late – so it was dark outside. (This was before I learned about the greatness of early morning running). I figured, what the heck – let me give the treadmill a try. So, down to the basement I went.

I had to admit – it was great! Instead of wearing layers of clothes, watching for sliding cars, being visible to those cars – I had on shorts and got in a great workout. Hmmm, maybe there was something to this treadmill thing after all!

Now, I still love to run outdoors – and always will if I can. But, I've learned that there are days that just scream – "Go downstairs to your friendly treadmill". And, like a best friend – it's always there for me!

I'm on my second treadmill now – and it's a lot fancier than my first one. I love it! And, I love knowing on those wind-blowing, below 0 days, I can still get in a great workout. I am so grateful that my husband talked me into that first one.

Be Sure You Can Be Seen

Another one of the best pieces of advice that I can give you is to make sure that oncoming cars can see you.

If you find yourself running in the early morning or late evening when it's dark out – make sure that you are wearing some sort of reflective clothing.

Running shoes are now made with some sort of reflective material – but it's usually not enough to make you visible as you should be.

They make all kinds of nifty reflective things now!

The most popular is the reflective vest. They are lightweight and most are made with some sort of moisture wicking material.

One of my favorites is the reflective arm/leg bands. I use mine around my ankles. I love them – you really don't even know you have them on. Now, they even make them with LED lights – which make you even more visible.

Reflective jackets are a great thing to have. I've got a lightweight one and one made for colder weather. If it's a day when you're going to wear a jacket anyway – one that is totally reflective is a great thing to have.

However, the reflective item that I use the most would be my reflective cap. It's totally fluorescent, glow in the dark yellow. It even has an LED blinking light on the back if I want to use it. I wear a cap everyday when I run anyway, so it's really convenient to just put this one on when it's dark.

As far as caps go, I've even seen ones that have a headlight on them. There are headlamps that are on a band that go on your head like a headband – or around your cap.

There are many ways to be reflective – just make sure that you are.

Just remember in your running – be safe!

Chapter 22 - My Incredible Support System

I would not have been able to have this great running life if it were not for the support of my wonderful husband, Bob. For almost all of the years that I've been running, he's been right there supporting me all the way.

There was a bunch of us that would travel out of town a few times a year to races. Either there and back or overnight. Their significant others and Bob would see us off and then be there at the finish with our "stuff". This was our running bags with dry clothing, shoes, and whatever else we thought we'd need at the end of the race. So, they became affectionately known as our "stuff holders"!

It's a lot to ask of a person to basically be bored to tears when they are waiting for their significant others to finish a race. If it was a short race, such as a 5K, I wasn't too bad. But, usually, if we traveled somewhere, the race was usually a 10K or longer. This meant an hour or more of waiting. And, if it was a marathon – you're looking at 4 hours and more.

Some of the races we attended with others, Bob and the other "waiters" would get breakfast to take care of some of the time. And, at some races, they would be able to see us on the course and offer support. But, there were many races, where there was nothing for them to do but wait.

My wonderful husband has always been a trouper. Even races where we traveled out of town by ourselves, he's never complained about the wait. And, most of the races are 2 hours or more for me to finish. Luckily, most races now have a shuttle to the start, so he can at least stay in the room and meet me later.

Throughout the years, Bob has backed me up all the way. Just a few of the places that we've gone for races are: Virginia Beach, Fort Lauderdale,

Washington, D.C., Orlando, and many more. He never says a word when I plan a "destination" race. He just drives me wherever I plan something.

He's always there at the end of my races with dry clothes and a drink. There are a couple of races where he's even had me a Pepsi when I most needed it! He loves to buy me things at the expos before larger races - I love that!

Whenever we are on vacation, Bob knows that I have to get my run in before we do anything else. There's never a question about it. He just asks me how long I need to run that day and what time I want to go out.

We built a restaurant about 10 miles from our house in 2000. He even put a shower in a building out back so that I could run to work and have a place to shower. How wonderful is that!

He is so good to me and I am so thankful for that. I can't imagine living with a spouse that is not supportive of my running.

If you feel that you're family members are not supportive of your running, sit down with them. Let them know why you run. Explain to them how important it is to you and how much you need their support. I'm sure that will help.

Support is important to your running – make sure everyone knows.

Conclusion

Well, that's my running story. I love my running –
and I love the places that it's taken me! I hope that
you've enjoyed my story and if you are a runner
already – I hope that my tips for staying out on the
roads will help.

See you out on the roads! As I always say –

Run Happy!

Resources

http://www.RunnerForLife.com   Sign up for my FREE weekly newsletter

http://www.RunAMileThisMonth.com   FREE training schedule for running your first mile

http://www.TheStreakingRunner.com   Follow me on my blog

http://www.budurl.com/RunA5K   A wonderful total program for beginning runners

http://www.budurl.com/runningbook My ebook on Kindle for beginning runners

http://www.RunningForBeginnersGuide.com My audio for beginning runners - what to do and what you need

http://FirstMarathonTips.com A great training program for running your first marathon http://www.budurl.com/GallowayOnRunning A must have book for all runners

http://www.budurl.com/RunningUntil100 A book for runners to stay running for life

http://www.budurl.com/Forerunner A great running GPS watch

 http://www.budurl.com/RunningID   Identification for runners

Dedication

A Tribute To The Man Who Taught Me How To Run – My Daddy

After I finished this book, my Daddy lost his 3 year battle with cancer. He fought a good hard fight up until the end – but I feel he just got tired.

I've always been a Daddy's Girl (even though I'm 50+ years old) and not ashamed to tell it. So, it's been a really rough time – but I'm remembering all the good times.

And, one of the best things is that my Dad is the one who got me running – and very early. When I was little, Daddy and I would go out in the evening and do 1 – 1/2 miles around our neighborhood. This was in the days before fancy running gear. So, it was just me in my P.F. Flyers. But, around the neighborhood we went.

Daddy even kept a log of our runs. How far and the time it took us. Those runs with my Dad were special to me. It was our time for him to hear about my day – and we just had fun being out there with each other.

I'm not sure how long we kept doing it – but eventually I guess the teen-age years took over and we didn't run anymore. I always wonder what would have happened to my running if I had kept it up.

Much of the person and runner I am today came from my Dad. He was also a very positive person his whole life. Even when his cancer came back he would always be positive and just say that "you have to play the cards that life deals you".

Daddy always had a lot of energy and was always doing something around the house. Even after he retired, there was always something he was doing. He was just not one to sit down for very long. I have definitely inherited this from him.

Mom and Daddy owned a retail clothing store for over 40 years. They worked side by side all that time. Watching them work together has helped me – I also work with my husband at our restaurant. I just hope that some of his business savvy has rubbed off on me.

Both of my parents instilled in me a sense of independence. Couple this with my being an only child and I think that's why I'm a long distance runner. I don't mind being by myself and you need to be able to like being alone if you're going to be out on the roads for 3+ hours.

They always supported my running. When I finished my first marathon, Mom and Daddy had traveled to the race so that they could be there when I finished. I'll never forget Daddy saying, "You look better after you finish a marathon than you do when you finish a 3-miler".

Daddy was a wonderful man and I'll miss him and his support in everything I do. And, that includes my running. Thank you, Daddy, for getting me out the door to run all those years ago!

www.ingramcontent.com/pod-product-compliance
Lightning Source LLC
Chambersburg PA
CBHW070158290526
45789CB00002B/820